I0405369

Nursing
Raw and Uncut

DISCLAIMER

Table of Contents

Introduction

There is often no place that nurses can go to unburden their hearts, or seek healing for themselves, except to a fellow nurse. For all those who have had the privilege of being cared for by a nurse, here in this book is a glimpse of their world.

We believe knowledge of a people and their perspective can change our world. This banter we offer in these pages is fun, and our purpose is to let it bring healing to our often unappreciated vocation. May this book bring laughter to our tired and often tried nerves. To all the nurses out there, this one's for you. But most of all, it is for those who have had a one-sided perception of what nurses really do.

We hope you enjoy our "unfiltered" humor. This banter is for the lightest of hearts. It is in no way, shape, or form a mockery of the sick or disabled. It is simply therapy for nurses. We also hope to bring awareness to those who often have a skeptical view of what goes on behind closed curtains. These are stories that nurses have lived. Some lives we encounter touch our hearts and remain with us forever. They are the driving force that keeps us returning to our profession as nurses. Unfortunately, there are also those patients who leave a long-lasting tart taste in our mouth, and for them there is no buffer! We hope this will shed light on our hard work, which often goes unrecognized at times.

How does it all begin? Who can forget! The journey of becoming a registered nurse is daunting. The fear of the unknown is scarier than our very first nursing class. It is only when we unite with others who share the same mission that we can feel at ease. Nursing students probably form the greatest bond as a group that you will ever come across. We also share the same uncensored sense of humor. It is where and how we shape our nursing sisterhood.

During the next few years together we begin to learn everything, from muscles and bones to medications we never thought of before, or even worse, where we have to give them. Just when we begin to build confidence, it is slowly put to the test when we encounter our first clinical instructor. Dressing in our nurse's uniform and purchasing our first stethoscope become so surreal. Then there is the moment we select our first pair of white Dansko nursing clogs, which in cost are roughly equivalent to one of our nursing books!

Anticipating our first day of clinical practice with fellow nurses for our morning huddle is exciting. We are now set free to care for real human beings as opposed to manikins from lab classes. Do you nurses out there remember bathing your first patient? Learning how to tuck the bed sheets and face the opening of the pillow case away from the door? The rationale of making the perfect bed free from wrinkles still stayed with us, adding to the neat appearance the perfect pillow case conveyed. Ironically, our future as nurses from this seemingly perfect façade was just a cover-up for the imperfect world we were about to enter.

Even scarier is our first realization that our clinical instructor is hovering behind our every move, expecting us to interact naturally with our patient. This time it is not the plastic, silent manikin that doesn't talk back. Rather, it is the almighty patient whose needs supersede everyone else's. That's right, we are not preparing hamburgers or stocking shelves—this is real human contact—the most frightening experience one could ever imagine.

Soon the time comes for us to venture out on our own, proudly gathering the bath items for our patient. We are now ready to embark on an unforgettable journey. Our emotions begin to shift swiftly when our perfect bath takes a sudden turn for the worse. Without notice, feces expel out of the patient's behind and land right on the nurse's shiny white Dansko's and we stand there horrified while our resident begins to yell at us wanting to know what's taking us so long . . . we are tortured with the repetitive thought as to why we ever chose this profession! There is nowhere to run, we are surrounded by the most putrid smell, and we try holding back our dry heaves to no avail. No classroom task can prepare our nose to adjust to all the new smells we will begin to encounter throughout our career from episodes like this one.

Nurses go above and beyond on a daily basis to provide excellent care, and they give the utmost respect to their patients. We are the most compassionate group of individuals you will ever encounter. *A unique group unlike any ever conceived.* Being a nurse is a calling that only other nurses can convey and understand. It means that we put our life on the line in the pursuit of protecting others, while our own may be at risk. We are an extraordinary selection of people, united not by color or gender but by the empathy and compassion that bind us. We protect and serve a growing population from all walks of life on a daily basis. Without judgment, we deliver care with pride to complete strangers, no matter what their ailments are.

Nurses are the first-line defenders of life, from its earliest stages to the very last moments when we become the sole presence at the end of life's journey. When life is at its most fragile, nurses are the ones who provide mercy to the afflicted. We wear coats of many colors, easing suffering, consoling those in despair, and advocating for the voiceless, just to mention a few. Often, we take upon our hearts the burdens of many. Weighed down with grief, we take on the woes of our patients and their families.

Nurses are the front-runners who treat patients without discrimination, exposing themselves to unknown pathogens that are highly contagious, yet keeping a smile on their faces. Blood, the constant lifesaving fluid that courses through our veins to bring forth nutrients and natural air to our bodies, can be the most dangerous avenue for fatal diseases. Through contaminated blood, a nurse can contract serious illnesses such as Human Immuno Deficiency Virus (HIV), Hepatitis, and other blood-borne pathogens. There are also the myriad of patients that present with sepsis—their contaminated blood can also be a source of contagion. The list goes on and on. Every nurse at one aspect of their profession or another has come in contact with contaminated or tainted blood. The methods of transmission are many, and cannot all be discussed within the context of this book. However, we are constantly faced with risk of exposure at any given time.

Some are very obvious, and other forms of contagion are subtle or unknown. Here is a glimpse of an incident that a nurse we spoke to recalled. When she was assisting with the insertion of a central venous catheter, the physician inserting it accidentally hit an artery in the groin and blood propelled into the air, almost entering the nurse's eyes. Discontinuing PICC lines, Central Venous Catheter Lines, is often a nurse's responsibility, and assisting in intubation, especially with a patient presenting with bleeding varices, poses another risk. Emptying of post-operative drains such as Hemovacs and Jackson-Pratt drains are also noteworthy as being procedures that put nurses at risk. Nurses come into contact with contaminated laundry and underpads stained with blood or other possible infectious materials. The soiled materials may also contain sharp objects, which can cut through the skin. Sharps objects include needles, scissors, blood tubes, and many more.

Most of us have broken skin, especially on our hands from the inevitable and frequent hand-washing. Therefore, contaminated blood can come in contact with that skin. In addition, time and time again, blood can suddenly splatter on our face after we draw blood from a patient. At times there is no escape from the unexpected blood and body fluids that can splash into our eyes, nose, lips, mouth, or onto our broken skin.

Most people shield themselves from any possible source of contagion, especially during flu season. Nurses have no shield; in fact, wearing protective equipment such as gowns and gloves, unless seriously warranted, can be very offensive to patients. We would never want them to feel bad about themselves, right? So when each and every one of us has had someone cough right in our face while starting an intravenous line, there's nothing we can do except maybe hold our breath for a minute. Let's face it, we are nurses, not deep-sea divers. Then what?

Yup, next, our worst fear becomes a reality. Upon returning to work the following day, we are greeted by a large sign on that same patient's door displaying the word "STOP." That same person had apparently been brewing a nasty infection that was sprayed right into our face. So now we're paranoid, right? We start taking zinc and Vitamin C in the hopes that we don't get our whole household sick. However, we better not call in sick the next day or we will have a lot to answer for, in more ways than one. In the blink of an eye we can be floated as a punishment to an unfamiliar unit upon our return. We can also find ourselves working most of the holidays to come. In truth, nurses spend most of their holidays with total strangers, while the patients' families are home celebrating. We provide care that most people couldn't fathom doing even for their closest relatives.

Surely, nursing is not for the faint of heart. Who do you know who would digitally disimpact someone for the sake of relief? To actually insert your finger into someone's anus and chip away at the hardened stool that refuses to pass on its own is an art that has been bestowed on us. Who would be willing to get scratched and spat on while trying to save a life and still remain composed? We are more than the glorified help, even though we're repeatedly called to fulfill unnecessary tasks like fluffing a pillow and reorganizing a room while other patients' cardiac alarms are sounding. If we leave a patient suddenly in a hurry, then we are considered rude and will be reported.

In fact, we are not allowed to tell any patient that their needs are not a priority, however minor. We certainly cannot break HIPAA (Health Insurance Portability and Accountability Act). Nurses have lost their licenses for unintentionally violating the patient's confidentiality. You simply cannot tell the patients who keep calling you the real reason their needs aren't a priority. Nurses can't say that the patient in the room next door is having a heart attack.

The truth is that nurses are sometimes treated as the patient's one-on-one personal assistant. Forget about the other seven patients who have their own issues that only the nurse can attend to. It doesn't matter, from the patient's perspective, that we are very educated and hold multiple degrees. It simply boils down to customer service and whether their stay at the hospital "Hilton" was satisfactory or not. Managers will immediately confront the nurse if there is any type of patient complaint. There have been many complaints against nurses from an array of "frequent flyers" who, let's just say, demand certain narcotics by name. For instance, if the patient is ordered narcotics to be given every four hours and the patient requests it sooner, we are considered offensive if we don't comply. Nurses are still—far too often—treated like dirt. *It makes no sense!*

Yet the actual background of the average nurse ranges from Doctor of Nursing Practice, Nurse Practitioner, Bachelor, Master, and Associate degrees. Nurses also hold various certifications, such as Certified Registered Nurse Anesthetist, Critical Care Nurse Certification, Advanced Cardiovascular Life Support, Pediatric Advanced Life Support, Neonatal Critical Care Nurse, Cardiac Medicine, and Cardiac Surgery and Certified Emergency Nurse. The varied nursing degrees are endless and cannot all be included. We don't look for praise for performing our job, but a little respect from time to time would go a long way!

Unfortunately, nurses are threatened at times and forced to work under intimidation and have to remain silent about it, whether the behavior comes from the patients themselves or the patients' family members. This intimidation and harassment, one would assume, cannot manifest itself in the center of healing and bringing forth wellness, but surprisingly it is at times constant, nevertheless. It starts at the beginning of the shift. We are badgered by family members of patients during change of shift report exchange which lasts maybe ten to fifteen minutes. Families interrupt us during report and literally accost us with insignificant demands. In addition, during the change of shift, vital information has to be handed over to the upcoming nurse to aid in the care of the patient. Sadly, there are no limits set by management. So these families of patients become *de facto* supervisors because if the nurse doesn't do what they ask at the second they ask it, the nurse will be reported.

The harassment does not abate until the nurse has paused in her report to straighten the wrinkled bedding for their family member. But it doesn't end there. As soon as the nurse on shift enters the patient's room to begin her assessment, families are requested to step out in order to afford the nurse the opportunity to thoroughly, and without interruption, examine the patient. Very often, the family blatantly refuses and openly stares the nurse down throughout her exam. Thus, in the midst of critical thinking and managing a variety of very challenging conditions singlehandedly, you are harassed by both families and patients. The public needs to recognize the skill level of nurses and that we deserve to be treated with courtesy. The respect nurses had in the past has somehow transformed over the past few years into hostility and aggression.

However, the air of suspicion that hovers among families of patients we care for is absurd. We understand there may be some underlying guilt people feel about not tending to their loved ones prior to their hospitalization, but may we remind you that the nurse is not the one to take it out on? Nurses are providing education, monitoring changes in vital signs, consulting with physicians and other healthcare providers, establishing treatment plans, observing changes in body systems and addressing them quickly to prevent any further serious medical emergencies. In addition, we deliver medications and monitor their side effects, feed patients, bathe them, and assist with diagnostic procedures.

We spend a great deal of time answering the many questions by families, even though those same questions were already answered by the previous nurse. Nurses are amazing multitaskers because they know the correct order of prioritization. Patients and their families should keep in mind that there probably was a valid reason why their nurse took a while coming to clean their bedside table. They were probably helping someone breathe who was unable to manage their own airway. A nurse is only one person and it's important to realize we are doing our very best. This is the case even though we are chronically understaffed, of course, but we're not even allowed to tell a patient that. We also cannot tell a patient that Cardiopulmonary Resuscitation (CPR) is being performed in the room next to them because that's against the privacy law.

On the other hand, we nurses have that special touch that soothes just about any ailment with a back massage. (We just make sure we warm up that lotion!)

Trust us, nurses would rather straighten sheets or deliver a hot cup of tea instead of losing the battle of saving lives to the hands of death. Not all medical interventions are a promise to maintain and sustain life. Nurses see life fade away in an instant before their very eyes. We console families at the bedside, contact organ donation centers, and prepare bodies for their final transport. Moments later, we answer the call bell only to apologize for taking too long delivering whatever was requested an hour prior, while still maintaining a positive attitude. Let the Therapy Session begin!

Chapter 1

R.E.S.P.E.C.T

Nurses can relate to the feeling that comes over us when code blue is announced through the loudspeakers. This unwelcome announcement is never a good sign, especially when it happens on our way to punch off the clock. Its aftereffect is like a hovering stigma that almost always precedes how our next twelve hours will be played out. The adrenalin begins without a caffeine induction. In an instant, we nurses are there, at that bedside, multitasking, doing what we do best. Often amidst the chaos that this particular emergency brings, the requests of the other unsuspecting patients do not abate. It's not a job that comes with predictable outcomes, but it's a job we do our best at, mustering a combination of skills—some taught, many acquired with experience and our own ingenuity. We begin to save the life that once emerged in the midst of joy, now fading into a state that we cannot battle with. Nurses are the ones who are there before doctors have had a chance to evaluate and assess.

The race to save lives, and the awareness of its fragility, is constantly before us and ultimately gives nurses the impetus to live life to its fullest. We are there as firsthand witnesses to life's end as a part of our daily work. We are not shelf-stockers, bank tellers, nor are we food service employees. That is not to minimize the importance of other career choices. We are simply making a point about the focus of the work we do: Nurses hold lives in their very hands. When new life enters this world, the ability of the newborn to thrive depends on the touch and care of a nurse. Lives that are in need of healing, that are broken, traumatized, poisoned, and sickened, all of them rely on the same hands that once were there when they first entered into the world. Nurturing is our norm, but we will change our demeanor in an instant when that patient decides to put themselves in harm's way. Yet, we are also very versatile and have to quickly adapt to the ever-speeding change of events on the spot. Tax preparers know the newest tax laws. In the same way, we as nurses know the newest algorithms that will save a life.

Everyone should feel blessed if they have a nurse in the family. It is sort of like having your own triage line that you can call anytime day or night! With that said, the next time you see a nurse and think to yourself "boy, she is kind of rude" or look at her sitting there drinking coffee, remember, she probably just lost a patient that she had been taking care of for a few days, or she could have worked the entire day supporting her patient's well-being whilst she missed her own children's breakfast, lunch, and dinner. Yes, we do drink coffee, because not only is it filling when we are starving to death, but it also gives us another burst of energy for our next round of turning and positioning our patient.

Have you ever wondered what that nurse was doing sitting behind the nurse's station? Well, here is a brief description of a day in the life of a nurse behind the scenes. Yes, we do sit to fill out charts because ergonomics tells us to do so. Did you know that ergonomics is part of nursing orientation? Back injuries are not allowed in the nursing profession even though we lift human bodies and equipment incessantly. Moreover, our bodies are forced into unnatural positions when lifting and hoisting human beings who are two to three times our size. No class can prepare your muscles for the effects of having to turn and position a patient every two hours. No wonder nurses suffer chronic back pain, multiple disc deformities and degenerations, to name a few. Many nurses at some point in their careers will suffer the aftermath of lifting heavy patients. But we don't dare mention that we have a back problem or call in as a result of a back injury. All hell will break loose on our unit and we definitely will feel like a criminal defending herself from a crime she didn't commit. Most nurses eventually give up and work under very painful conditions for which there may be no remedy to avoid the harassing scrutiny of having to defend their "sick time," or the mounds of paperwork that they have to present in order to get reprieve from an inevitable back problem. Nurses are often the sacrificial lambs who as a result of an act of mercy end up with an incurable condition. Sadly, not only do they suffer but their families do, as well.

Nurses chart like there is no tomorrow. Why? Because before a patient can receive their cough medicine, we have to check the order to see when they had it last, chart what kind of cough they have, not to mention the color and consistency of their secretions. In addition, it must be evaluated whether or not they are able to clear their own airway or not. Last but not the least, we must sign on to the computer at their bedside after entering three different passwords in order to scan their wristband. The nurse's station is not a hideout—rather, it's a spotlight, and we really don't want to be center stage. Who knows better than us that no one wants our autograph, except when it's on a written warning?

The nurse's station holds vital information. For example, this is where the cardiac rhythms display on monitors along with vital signs and oxygen levels. Yes, it's the nurse, not the cardiologist, who monitors the cardiac rhythms for the duration of the patient's hospital stay. We diligently monitor the various waveforms and report critical abnormalities in the patient's vital signs, preventing any further worsening problems that may ensue. The cardiac monitors with distinct sounds that stays in our psyche long after our shift is over.

Oh, by the way, did we mention that nurses work twelve hour shifts, and no, they don't get to have a "closed" sign to place in front of them so they can go to lunch? A nurse cannot just go to the bathroom when the need arises, either, because just when nature calls, the patient rings. Without hesitation the patient becomes top priority and we must not let them ring their call bell twice, lest they call us negligent. It is definitely bad customer service that we must avoid. After all, we don't want to be the main highlight of the infamous patient's callback or reported during the morning rounds led by the nurse manager, rounds that are in actuality really a follow-up on how we have treated patients.

Sadly, we are not the enemy and we are tired of being viewed as one. We are the unsung heroes who continually hold every life as precious and worthy of being defended. The world is changing at a fast pace and we continue to keep up without extra help or raises. Raises, you may ask? Yes. No matter what we make, it's not enough. Court reporters, sales agents, mail carriers, dental hygienists and fitness instructors, to name a few, get paid equal to a nurse or slightly more. So why is the concept of our pay so hard to conceive when we work with bodily fluids on a daily basis? We are constantly at risk, whether it's the confused patient who puts us at risk for being stuck by a contaminated needle because they keep squirming while we try to obtain lab specimen, or the HIV patient who needs an intravenous line. In our opinion, we don't get paid enough. The saddest thing is, corporations and small businesses are known for doing everything they can to prevent raises for nurses that are long overdue. We wish we knew why that was, considering nurses are the ones making the money for the hospital. They are the ones at risk, not the CEO who frequents business luncheons multiple times per week.

Yes, staffing is a huge issue in nursing today, as everyone knows. Nurses are not allowed to speak of it because then the patients' families and residents would worry. We certainly cannot have that! Meanwhile, we can't keep up with the demands of all our patients because we now perform tasks of the ancillary departments; such as the Respiratory department, EKG department, X-ray, Laboratory and Pharmacy. Either way, it is a doomed situation for us. Let's not forget the unfounded complaints that keep coming against us, too. One famous complaint is that it took too long for us to bring that extra blanket, or that we did not clean up that spilled glass of water for the fifth time in a timely manner.

Yet, when the world sleeps, we are vigilant, working long, arduous shifts at times without breaks. Every cell of our bodies is working against our own circadian rhythms. Think of the circadian rhythms as our sleep-wake cycle. What happens when it becomes disrupted? Health problems can arise from the interference of our natural body rhythms, including chronic illnesses such as metabolic disorders that can lead to obesity, diabetes mellitus, hypothyroidism, and hyperthyroidism. Also, hypertension, inflammatory issues, and the constant feeling of being jet-lagged could ensue. To stay alert, nurses force themselves to stay awake with bottomless cups of coffee. Therefore, it's no surprise that they end up with palpitations by morning. In addition, nurses continuously snack on unhealthy foods that create unwanted side effects.

Not only are we scrutinized by the many unstable personalities that belong to the families of patients, we constantly have to stop our patient care to hear about all the people in a patient's family who have careers as nurses and doctors. Well, friends, we are not intimidated by this in any way, shape, or form. By the time our exhausting shift has ended we are even made very aware that a family member holds a very high position as a home health aide. We are not denigrating the importance to the world of home health care, but listen, we are critical care nurses who can handle a few runs of ventricular tachycardia or placing a bipap (Bi-level positive airway pressure) machine on someone without being told to do so! Those procedures require a high level of skill that deserves to be recognized.

Please, attention must be paid to this truth: **We treat all our patients equally regardless of their socio-economic background.** Let's not forget that it is the nurse who is in the forefront of locating translators to suit the needs of foreign-speaking patients. Nurses are also instrumental in preventing the substance abusers who are in withdrawal from further harming themselves. We go to great lengths to protect our patients from pulling out their intravenous lines while getting cursed out and criticized by those same patients. We also provide care for the incarcerated patients who are hospitalized, despite their having committed crimes against children. Nurses care for the patient with tuberculosis while the rest of the world fears them. Almost half of the patients hospitalized today are admitted with some sort of blood-borne pathogen, and yes, we still care for them without prejudice, and provide them with whatever their needs may be. Need we say more? Think of the correctional nurses who without discrimination come to the aid of the criminal who previously committed the heinous crime of murdering a helpless elderly woman. Or the medical surgical nurse who has more patients than their rolling computer can keep up with.

It is the critical care nurse who deserves more recognition than the nurse's aide who delivered a pitcher of water, as this example shows. A patient after a three-night stay in the intensive care unit recovered without complications and was transferred to the step down unit because he was doing so much better. During his stay the diligent critical care nurse utilized every intervention possible to prevent the patient from being intubated and placed on a ventilator. With a firm and purposeful demeanor, she repeatedly encouraged the patient to take deep breaths, use breathing equipment, percussion, change positions, go through inhalation medication treatments-- basically providing one-on-one attention to him. After his third day of arriving at his new unit, he had nothing but complaints about the nurse who had saved his life. He insisted she was rude and demanding. When this patient received his callback to evaluate his stay, his only positive remark was that the friendly nurse's aide provided him with a fresh water pitcher!

While the critical care nurse may only have "one" patient, she is multitasking and delivering a variety of acute crucial interventions: Balancing the treatments and medication of the regime, monitoring wave forms of the patient who has an intra-aortic balloon pump, continuous hemodynamic monitoring, and balancing transducer lines at the phlebostatic axis correctly, and relaying the information appropriately to the doctors to receive the correct medication dosages, in the attempt to maintain cardiac output. That critical care nurse also knows when and which lab specimens need to be obtained. She also obtains arterial blood samplings and titrate vasopressor agents.

Have you ever wondered why the critical care nurse stands and stares at the monitor while flushing an intravenous line to maintain patency? Her relaxed expression is not one of a lack of motivation or laziness. Might we add that she is not watching the patient's TV from afar while absentmindedly delivering medication? Rather, she is observing the monitor for a number. Pulmonary capillary wedge pressure is the pressure measured by wedging a pulmonary catheter with an inflated balloon into a small pulmonary arterial branch. This is performed for the purpose of obtaining a direct number that reflects hemodynamic stability. The procedure in itself is very serious and can be life-threatening. It can lead to serious arrhythmias, thrombosis, infection, rupture of the pulmonary artery, pneumothorax, and bleeding.

So the next time anyone feels ready to judge a seemingly "bored" nurse, thinking she's not doing anything but standing around, think twice, because her brain synapses are probably firing off like the Fourth of July fireworks. The only difference is—there's no picnic going on!

Chapter 2

Old vs. New

Every nurse began somewhere and we all remember that horrifying moment when we had to give our first patient report. And of course, we have to give it to the "all-knowing" nurse who's never forgotten as much as a patient's name, much less where the patient lives and their social habits. Experienced nurses are the ones that hold it together. They are the calm and collected ones who deliver when issues arise. They are the nurses you want on your team.

Sometimes you may encounter a seasoned nurse who may be so burnt out from thirty-plus years of nursing, she simply has not an ounce left in her to train another new employee. But for the seasoned nurse, having the patience to train the new nurse will be beneficial in the long run. When an emergency occurs, it will not be only the seasoned nurse running to the "rescue" as the one and only responder. Properly orienting the new nurse will only make the seasoned nurse's job as the "responder" easier. When she arrives because of those rapid responses that are frequently announced overhead, the experienced nurse will not have to perform most of the interventions alone.

Why do nurses tend to "eat" their young? This term is commonly used among nurses. It refers to the stern treatment that some senior or more experienced nurses have toward the new nurse. We never really understood the rationale behind it. At times, the competent nurse may respond to a newbie with a stern attitude if a brand new nurse with no experience is overconfident. Some newbies do convey a "know it all" attitude which impedes teaching, and can be a roadblock to success as a competent practitioner. On the other hand, will giving someone a shortcut or advice somehow lessen the power of the trainer or preceptor?

We need to teach the new nurses who are starting their careers, who think they know everything, how to assess a patient in "real life." Nursing assistants who have transitioned to being registered nurses do have a predisposition to think they already know everything. Of course, they don't. The thing is, once we've entered the other side, it's a whole new game out there. We may have had time long ago to relax and chat with our patients while providing active daily living assistance to them. Not anymore. Now, we are actually responsible for that patient and if anything happens to them, it's our butt on the line. We may not have the same amount of time we once had because now our patient load comes with many more activities and interventions.

Time management is of the essence now, and newbies must pay attention to the veteran nurse who is trying to teach them. Nursing school does not prepare us for the sharky waters we must fight in to stay alive. Our advice to new nurses is to listen, pay attention, and if you don't know something, speak up. Lives depend on your skill assessment and things can go very wrong when you overlook certain symptoms.

New Nurse Report Fails

You have to love those reports from new nurses that begin with "I just picked this patient up four hours ago." Okay, so right there that nurse is simply saying that she has absolutely no knowledge of this patient and please don't ask her any questions. Seriously, people, in this situation seasoned nurses can become, well, let's just say, not so nice!

Another example is, "He was fine an hour ago." That has to be the worst thing a new nurse can say in a report. Yes, things happen very fast in the medical field but rigor mortis is not one of them! You simply try to refrain from laughter when the nurse states that she removed the patient's non-re-breather so the patient could eat dinner and never supplemented oxygen via nasal prongs. The nurse delivers this with such a straight face, like why are we so concerned she removed the patient's mask? Well, considering the patient's blue skin doesn't go well with the green hospital gown, we think the mask should be put back on! The patient who requires one hundred percent oxygen to survive has now had her air basically taken away. Not only was the oxygen removed, but so was the oxygen sensor on her finger which displayed her oxygen levels. When the finger probe was finally reapplied by the experienced nurse, the saturation was sixty percent, and that is not compatible with life. Nurses are very happy to see numbers above ninety-four, which is roughly the average norm.

We might read the newbie's stat transfer report and find it merely consists of what the patient ate for dinner, their last bowel movement, and what they like to be called. Then we receive the patient to find them in an unresponsive state, soon to be resuscitated, or on arrival we notice the so-called stable patient has a mouth full of vomit. In addition, their skin is pale and clammy with no intravenous access. Now, these are a few minor details that we as experienced nurses would appreciate. We could care less about where they live or what they ate for dinner!

You just can't make this stuff up.

The best new nurse report fail is when we are told the patients' blood sugar was twenty-five and the newbie gave them a snack. Meanwhile, we are thinking about the last patient we had with that same blood sugar. They were unresponsive! The only sugar they were consuming was through their intravenous line.

Still, we can't get over the time when the patient's heart rate was one hundred and sixty and we were told "Oh, that always happens when they ambulate to the bathroom." In actuality, we are wondering why the patient is even out of bed. Okay, now we are predicting a fall because we are sure that blood pressure is dropping as we speak. Cardiac output can only last so long when the heart is beating that fast in an eighty-year-old!

One report was received on an incoming patient that stated the patient had a *heparin drip* infusing, although reason was unknown. Shortly after receiving the patient, the newbie nurse actually had a *hespan drip* infusing in the attempt to expand the patient's volume to increase their blood pressure! So just because the medication bag has a letter H on it doesn't mean the new nurse shouldn't read the entire name!

New Nurse Humor

It's amazing when you help a code situation on a floor you are unfamiliar with and the staff can't figure out how to open their own crash cart. What's worse is when you call out for something and they run down the hall to get it, when all along it was in the cart next to them.

New nurses have a tendency toward tunnel vision. They can't chart and use the mouse to stop the telemetry alarms from sounding at the same time. Or for that matter understand why the lethal alarm is sounding.

Imagine overhearing a new charge nurse relaying information to the doctor over the phone requesting more beta blockers for her patient's new increase in heart rate. Like any seasoned nurse you offer a lending hand and begin to ask a few questions. When you discover the patient hasn't even been assessed yet, you venture down the hall to find this little elderly woman stuck in her bed rails. So really the hidden undertone here is, please check the patient first!

Some new nurses love the adrenalin rush while others simply avoid it at all costs. Performing CPR for the first time can be very frightening, especially when the new nurse is center stage, or pushing her first ampule of sodium bicarbonate while her hands are pleading for help. Everyone has to learn some time, but if she can't even open the box of atropine, it's probably best for her to hang in the back and record events.

It's actually amusing for the experienced nurse to watch their new preceptee entering the patient's isolation room without gathering all the supplies they will need beforehand. Then once they finally finish donning their isolation gown, gloves, and mask they realize they need a bunch of things. They stand in the doorway waiting for someone to pass so they can call out for the ten items they had forgotten. You really are trying to be nice, but what you want to do is throw them one at a time at her and tell her to stop being lazy and come out herself. This will only teach her in the future not to be a little princess expecting the red carpet treatment.

You can definitely decipher between a new nurse and an experienced nurse when they come in to receive report. The new nurse goes straight to the computer, refusing any verbal contact until she has read her SBAR, whereas the experienced nurse grabs a cup of coffee prior to any interaction. Then the experienced nurse is ready to talk, usually without writing or viewing any computers.

These are prime examples why seasoned nurses need to coddle their young, even though it may be frustrating at times teaching new nurses who think their way is best. It's important to remember once upon a time we were all once in their shoes. Think back to all the shortcuts you've learned over the years and how easy life became when you were busy with six or seven patients.

After a while, you can generally predict the course of illness and how it will play out. Your knowledge and early recognition is what saves lives. Knowledge is power. Don't be afraid to share it.

Chapter 3

Lithium For All

Dementia is a very lonely world that nurses can attest to from having witnessed it in patients. It's heartbreaking to be a bystander and see the painful loss families and their loved ones experience. We strive in every moment around them to create a sense of normalcy. It is an insidious disease that nurses know firsthand. There is a special attention we pay to these patients, spending time with them, encouraging and listening to their repeated fragmented stories. When the patient's family members go home, nurses become their friend, confidant, family member, and advocate. At times, we become the protector as they recall their painful past from years ago, or their consoler as they remember in their mind's eye their grief, searching for a deceased spouse or a child that preceded them. We give every ounce of our being to their service. "Attempt"--as it is professionally known--is "reorienting" an aging patient who is friend by day and foe by night when they "sundown." We continue to remind the patient where they are, in addition to the date and time. Unfortunately, when the sun goes down the patient turns into the dark version of themselves, hence the term "sun downing." It's an odd phenomenon, but it's as real as night and day.

The Sundown Syndrome is when our patient gets confused at night. The familiar words we know so well really mean they stay up all night kicking at any and everything, including us, with no end in sight. If and when we try to prevent them from harming themselves, we become the foe, viewed as their attacker who must be battled with throughout our shift--while we still have to maintain our professionalism. There usually isn't an armor that will protect against stool-filled finger nails, projectile spitting, or bodily fluids thrown at us. Knowing the condition of our patients' psyche, we expect them to pull off all their monitoring equipment and call us all kinds of unpleasant names. While they are at it, one can almost predict what's to come. They will accuse us next of trying to kill them. All the while they are attempting to paste feces all over our new scrubs, as we are only trying to save their life while ours is in danger.

Well, my friends, all these things do happen and yes, we do take it in stride and in good faith. God bless patients who suffer from dementia, but if we have to explain just one more time why there is a dog at the nurse's station smoking a cigarette, we're going to lose it!

What about the patient who suffers from hepatic encephalopathy? This condition can also create confusion and altered mental status changes. Another complication is the accumulation of toxic substances that build up in the intestines. The best way to help treat this underlying condition is to give laxatives.

Unfortunately, this will produce excessive amounts of diarrhea, our old-time favorite lactulose, the medicine that cleans you out in the name of cleansing out toxins! Leaving your patient, as some nurses call it, "in a pool of stool or a continuous code brown." Until their confusion begins to subside, you may find them later playing in it trying to create a Monet on their bed board!

There are also those patients who make us feel as if we're the crazy one by shift's end. It's not their fault they have no control over their brain synapses. At times, a nurse is not always sure which personality is presenting before them. The ability to interpret our world as we see it is different from those who live with these disorders. Their reality is distorted in an array of personalities that a nurse must sort out. Some patients can exhibit impulsivity in controlling their behavior, lack of empathy and arrogance, while others display absolutely no filter in their comportment.

It's most trying when patients think you are part of this big conspiracy to abduct them or they hear helicopters flying above, when in reality it is so quiet you can actually hear a pin drop. Yet, they are refusing their antipsychotic medications. There's no protection for nurses if the patient lunges at them. Many nurses have been attacked behind locked mental units and have actually returned to their same unit. *Nurses have this devoted sense of obligation to their patients.* Luckily, there are a huge variety of us that take on different callings.

On the other side of the spectrum, there's the patient who becomes psychotic of their own volition, whether it be drugs or alcohol. The next time you are abusing happy hour you may find yourself in some hospital room seeing hotdogs dancing on the ceiling and you will definitely need a good nurse on your side. That nurse either becomes the punching bag or means to an end of recovery. Still, nurses do not retreat, but join forces with their fellow nurses to bring the addicts back to a state of normalcy. At times this is done at a very expensive cost. Nurses are bruised, not only physically, but psychologically. Many contract life-threatening diseases from which there may be no remedy or support.

We are human beings and can only take so much in a twelve-hour shift. Nurses sometimes have to control their own filter. We may think things and have opinions and reactions, but we would never mention them.

In the morning after we've sustained a very trying shift, our psychiatric patient who refused to take her meds is now asking: "You got all my meds?" And we are tempted to answer, "Yeah, all except the lithium, I took that one!"

Whether the underlying cause of confusion was deliberate or not, we as nurses treat each and every patient as an entire being and not merely a symptom. They all require many different treatment plans and we adapt with ease to the six-foot-tall gentleman who is going through withdrawal and tries to flee, to the ninety-year-old woman with a stool as a weapon and a saucy mouth, or to the hypoxic patient who is sucking on the hub of their heparin-lock. We are the ones who, even after having been repeatedly "knocked down," will in turn return to become the anchor that saves a patient's ass. We just want them to remember we are here to save it, not kiss it.

Chapter 4

The Ugly Truth

Our nursing career has many advantages, although there is one major disadvantage. It is dealing with contaminated bodily fluids: blood, sputum, stool, urine, gastric contents, and wound drainage to name a few. There is a constant fear that lurks over a nurse whenever we have to empty drainage bags, surgical drains, or any other canister that had been used as collection device. The horrific thought of any little microscopic splatter crossing over into our eyes or even touching our skin is terrifying. The thought that maybe something might have touched us becomes our worst fear. In a state of panic we race to the sink to scrub and use alcohol on any possible surface that could have been exposed. At that moment we feel so isolated and frightened with the thought that we might have been invaded by an unknown pathogen that could mar our lives forever.

Not only is this vocation dangerous, it has a stinky side that we have to contend with. There are many pros and cons of being a nurse. We are here to tell you that unpleasant smells is something you never get used to. Our words are not of ridicule, but are of respect to those who continue to perform noble acts which sometimes goes unnoticed. With a face of compassion and understanding, we walk into the center of the fire, showing an air of respect and sympathy for those afflicted with these symptoms. Again and again, we come to their rescue, without judgment, and deliver.

Let's talk about the smell of feces. Nurses are the ones alerted when duty calls. We also manually help those who are not only constipated, but quite often, those who can't stop going. Either way, we are there with a straight face despite the fumes that are invading our nasal passages. Nurses at times are quite entertained by morbid jokes that only they can comprehend. We make jokes and have a weak stomach at times. But who wouldn't in this profession? Humor at its best is what keeps us sane when we are standing there covered with splatters of bright green vomitus while fighting our own dry heaves. Any situation becomes bearable when your coworker comes to your aid. It is only when another nurse comes in to clean feces with you, do you truly feel the support of another.

The next time anyone is bombarded by the odor of someone's flatus invading their senses, think of nurses. Nurses can only tolerate so much and there remain a few smells that can still jolt the most seasoned of nurses:

Top Ten Most Offensive Smells to Nurses

- Most nurses will agree that the most nauseating smell is from the gastrointestinal bleeds. It is the smell of a rotten egg that has been in ninety-degree weather for hours. No one can tolerate the pungent air that brings tears to the eyes. Yet we must not make a grimace, because it's not allowed. We are not only changing copious amounts of gelatinous bright red bloody stools every twenty minutes, we are also trying to maintain our composure.

- Clostridium Difficile is a spore-forming bacteria that overtakes intestines and attacks the lining producing frequent diarrhea. It has the most odorous smell that you will ever come across. Its sting leaves a long lasting odor all over you. It is like the long expected dam that broke with a vengeance. Any nurse can attest to this fact.

- We empathize with those patients who live with the daily battle of a non-healing wound. However, the odorous smell that emanates from the wound hovers over the nurse, way after she has left the confines of the room. It's unfortunate that air fresheners are prohibited in most medical facilities--the patient would most benefit as well.

- Who hasn't emptied the morning urinary catheter without getting that initial gust of ammonia scent, hot as the heat of the desert sun?

- The fishy vaginal odor that stems from a yeast infection combined with a cottage cheese-like discharge leaves no nurse with an appetite. No meal break for us today. Collect your own urine sample, please.

- The unpleasant aroma from the pseudomonas growing from the decaying wound or around tracheostomy sites leaves us feeling like we are in need of stat anti-emetics.

- Anyone, who has cleaned up copious amounts of vomitus can attest to the fact that they would rather be cleaning up a contaminated sewage spill. It is the most repugnant smell a nurse is faced with. Not only is it vile, it sometimes contains large chunks of food in its original form. Like, did they chew or what?

- Tube feed is a form of nutrition that is delivered through a nasogastric tube, for those who cannot take in any form of solids through their mouths. This provides a route directly to their stomach. If you ever had a child that vomited formula, this is the smell we are referring to.

- Let's not forget to talk about the body's waste system. Its excrement is a makeup of human waste matter that greets us in many shapes, consistencies, and aromas. Sometimes it's a form that resembles that of a human head or is as watery as the unending Nile.

- Flatus is a gas that is expelled through the intestinal tract and exits out the anus. Break wind, cut the cheese, rip one, poof, toot, whatever you call it, we don't want to smell it!

Nurses specialize in noxious odors, sticky unknown substances and contaminated body fluids on a daily basis. One inevitable mishap that can occur secondary to caring for "sick" patients may be our doom. For example, awareness must be brought to nurses who are faced with an acquired illness, secondary to cross-contamination. It is almost always the nurse's fault. That poor nurse will be criticized step by step for not ensuring all universal precautions per policy. However, universal precautions no matter how strictly followed are not a hundred percent protection for nurses. Management isn't there when the patients are sometimes flinging things at nurses. They will always consider this poor customer service, if the nurse raises their voices to the patients. But there are many forms of assault against nurses.

Consider the simple and well-known case of influenza. Patients at times knowing that they have the flu would still cough right in your face. Please, people, cover your mouth. But we really want to say, who taught you manners? Turn your head when you cough and cover your mouth. You are aiming your Methicillin Resistant Staphylococcus Aureus (MRSA) right in our face. We understand sometimes patients are so sick and cannot help it, but we have encountered many alert patients who feel the need to cough in our face. Yes, we say MRSA because most patients turn positive during their stay at the "Hilton."

The Icky Side of Nursing: Telling It Like It Is

Nurses cannot escape the endless ocean of bodily fluids that comes at them in all its glory. Whether it is projectile by mouth or down below, we are usually equipped, but can never arm ourselves enough for the unexpected nature of this profession. Yet we remain at our patient's bedside knowing very well that tomorrow we could be the ones who could be bitten by the same bug that we strive to destroy. Consider these truths:

- Nurses go above and beyond. We are the ones behind closed curtains when our patient cries out for the bed pan stat because they are having diarrhea.
- We are the ones, for the sake of helping someone breathe, will navigate with a suction tube through their nose or mouth to retrieve copious amounts of backed up phlegm.
- We are the ones inserting a nasal gastric tube while the patient is vomiting from what appears to be feces due to a blockage.
- We are holding pressure on an area that would not stop bleeding in patients on anticoagulants or blood diseases that cause profuse bleeding.
- We empty surgical drains that are filled with drainage: infectious pus, blood, or simply just contaminated serous fluid that has the potential of spraying into our eyes.

- We insert rectal catheters for the continuous mudslide that presents itself with certain illnesses.
- We change dressings to wounds of all depths and grades. Some are flesh-eating, some are due to vascular insufficiency. Regardless of the severity we are face-to-face with the drainage.

We have to prepare to pay close attention to all the above, because we will be required to chart every bodily fluid description we encounter, leaving out no detail.

Now, are there any nurses you know that are not lighthearted? Not likely. We can talk about bodily fluids while seated among family members at the dinner table. It is everyday conversation to us. It is not to offend anyone. It is simply what we are used to. Well, as they say, nursing is not for those with a weak stomach. For some of us, though, we put on a good attitude before patients and "exhale" when we can. We are only human—mortal beings whose wings are compassion and mercy.

Chapter5

Don't Bite The Hand That Feeds You

How many nurses out there have had thoughts of what they wish they could say to those annoying patients who simply harass them for the fun of it? These patients do this because they can. We have all been there. It's amazing the power that the call bell has in the hands of a patient. Like that sweet little old lady who initially resembles your grandmother and who is so cute at the beginning of your shift. Then, by three a.m., she becomes transformed into someone you have never met before. She becomes bowel-obsessed, asking for her "physic" repeatedly because she hasn't had a bowel movement in one whole day. Regardless of your heated prune juice and the multiple bed pan attempts, she then asks you to digitally assist in the evacuation of the hardened stool from her anus. Not so cute any more.

What about that patient who is surrounded by a party of family members laughing and eating Doritos? Now the patient claims their pain level is ten out of ten as soon as we introduce ourselves to them as their nurse. In an instant, the patient's laughter turns into a dramatized clenching of fists, body tremors, intense moaning, and complaints of how severe their pain is. Mind you, they then continue to stare at the clock whilst we administer their medicine, with a now calm expression on their face. While faithfully infusing their so-called needed pain medicine, they begin to question you as to when they are allowed to have the next dose!

There are also those patients who post selfies of themselves on social media enjoying the narcotics they had received. Weeks later, they complain to the callback team about how dissatisfied they were with the care given by the nursing staff. We do remember "those" patients and NO, they were never deprived of their pain medicine!

Another very common occurrence in the midst of caring for our patients is that, in our very busy schedules, we do our best to massage their backs before they retire for the night. It never fails when the first remark that seems to come out of their mouth is, the lotion is too cold. Usually, this is said in the most sarcastic and loud manner one could imagine. Regardless of our repeated attempts to warm it up, our efforts have failed us in the patient's mind.

Fellow nurses, don't you love it when incoming patient sitters walk in escorted by their own assistants carrying their heavy laptop bag? Upon entering the unit, they announce that they have a bad back and "don't do cares." Sitters are aides assigned to keep watch over a particular patient. Depending on their specific job requirements, they can help the patients with all their needs, including keeping them safe.

The sitter's exaggerated entrance is their proclamation that they are merely present to sit and do nothing. Never mind the very busy patient they have been assigned to who needs to be assisted on the bed pan every 15 minutes, or who is severely overweight and needs the assistance of several staff members. In the very next breath, the sitter accosts you to show them where to plug their computer and tells you they require a recliner to rest their aching back. "I'll tell you where you can plug it" is what we would really like to say. Then, towards the end of the shift, a miraculous healing happens—that same sitter is found scurrying out the door with her "heavy" laptop bag on her shoulder. She not only walks, but practically dances her way out of the unit so fast that one could almost envision sparks flying beneath her sneakers.

Simply Annoying Things

Truly, it takes a great amount of patience and fortitude to withstand the many forms of harassment that nurses endure.

- After our grueling twelve-hour shift we pack to go home, only to have our boss remind us of the mandatory Ebola training that is set to begin in the next few minutes.
- When drawing a patient's blood, they jerk their arm, causing blood to splatter in our face.
- Family members feel the need to call us repeatedly at odd hours of the night just to tell us the most basic methods of nursing care, such as "Do not forget to sit

my mother up when she is getting tube feeds."
Whoever heard of a person eating while supine?

- Family members also ask each nurse from each shift the same question to see if we are consistent. We know this—we know what they're up to.

- We all know how annoying it is when we are exiting an isolation room after we have asked our patient repeatedly if they needed anything else. As soon as we de-gown, they ask us for fresh ice water. Really?????

- Then consider the case of the eavesdropping patient—the one who complains that there is too much chatter at the nurses' station, only to turn down their television so they can listen. By the way, they add, "Keep the curtain open, I like to see what is going on out there."

- The patient who refused their routinely scheduled sleeping pill bitterly blames their nurse in the morning, saying that they hadn't slept a wink.

- How about the classic case of a patient who repeatedly soils the bed right after the nurse has given a complete and tedious bath with no assistance in sight?

- It also never fails that when we go into a patient's room to draw their blood, the first comment they make to us is that we shouldn't attempt it because no one has been successful.

- Many a time, we call doctors in the wee hours of the morning for orders and it's like we are interrupting King Arthur and his Knights having dinner at the Round Table. "I'm sorry to bother you, sir, like I have nothing better to do at this hour than be berated by you."

- Your patient's Clostridium Difficile explodes all over your "so-called" isolation gown and you are praying it didn't hit your face.

- Blood splatters all over every possible orifice imaginable after we perform the most frequent of tasks, which is obtaining blood from a patient's finger to check their blood sugar.

- The cardiac monitor continues to alarm because the high tech system cannot decipher between multifocal Premature Ventricular Beats and Ventricular Tachycardia.

- Above all, the most annoying occurrence that one can endure for twelve hours straight is that coworker who talks incessantly about themselves. We all have encountered a few of these "chatty Cathys" who enjoy hearing the sound of their own voices, rather than the cardiac alarms. They refuse to interpret correctly the loud hints that our inattention signifies.

After our pain and suffering comes to a welcomed end, we find ourselves trying to remove our previous thoughts of intubating her from our mind.

- As soon as we get our intubated patient settled, the family parades in and one can feel the aura of suspicion on their faces. Without words, they convey their displeasure at seeing their loved one on a ventilator. If looks could kill, we would exist no more. They honestly have no idea what we do behind closed curtains. If only they were there thirty minutes earlier, they would have seen their loved one struggling for every breath, while their heart rhythm was in and out of every lethal arrhythmia possible. They would have seen our mad rush to assemble a response team, administer medications, address cardiac symptoms, and place all the appropriate required lines for the stability of the patient. Now, with that said, without our astute interventions, their loved one would be no more. Perhaps a thank you would have been more appropriate? Eventually, when we exit the patient's room unscathed and think we're in the clear to begin charting our every move leading up to the most recent events, there the family are again. Just when we think we've heard it all, the patient's family asks if that patient can have a drink of water. We are thinking "Please forgive my rudeness, but do you not see that large tube wedged in their throat?" Patience, they say, is a virtue, and now is the time to remain calm.

- Introducing ourselves to the patient at the beginning of our shift can be trying. It never fails when credentials are literally thrown at us upon our kindly introduction. The famous response that sends any nurse rolling their eyes is when the patient refers to the fact that their cousin is a nurse or their wife's sister is a paramedic. Well, "Nice to meet you" is what we say but what we are really thinking is, "Good--let them take your ass home and care for you then!" Meanwhile, we are also thinking, "Boy it's going to be a long shift!

- If only our managers had the courage to defend us against those well-known troublemaking family members! Morale would be much better. Perhaps then when they need us to work an extra shift, we would!

- However, nothing tops the time when the family complained about the nurse who reiterated the visiting hours, only to have repercussions later. That nurse was spoken to and the family was sent a free lunch cart. Now this only says to the family "Feel free to harass your nurse and take over because rules do not really matter."

- Ten hours into our shift we finally get a chance to sit and eat our very cold dinner and our patient's heart rate tops one-hundred-eighty. The nerve!
- As evening approaches we begin to review our most recent orders and we discover a tube feed order that should have been started six hours earlier.
- We go in and measure our patient's nasogastric tube output to find it plugged and backed up onto our perfectly fresh and newly-changed linens.
- We come into work and discover our partner called in sick and we're floated a nurse who has absolutely no idea how to use the equipment in our area and won't stop texting.
- Nurses, have you in the call of duty, while entering a patient's room who is on isolation, been asked when you sneezed, "Are you sick?" in the most suspicious of tones, as if we have brought whatever bug we have to spread to this patient? Let's not reiterate that this patient is herself positive for influenza, and has been coughing all day. Nurses are not made of armor but at least nurses cover their mouths.
- Nothing is more annoying than entering a patient's room when they are supposed to be soundly sleeping and they sit bolt upright asking to be washed at three a.m.!

- As nurses we must deliver verbal reports to one another at the beginning and end of our shifts. This is a time that is very crucial because information is exchanged regarding current treatments, diagnosis, prognosis, plan of care, and history, among many other pieces of data. During this time we would appreciate it if we were not disturbed for insignificant things. It is like our happy hour. For the incoming nurses they have time to finish their coffee and for the outgoing nurses it is their long-awaited thirst that has been quenched after a long and grueling shift. Guess what? It never seems to fail that it is at that exact minute when most patients call out that have to move their bowels. Every time, it turns out that it was just some forced flatus. It's almost like they are giving us departing well wishes—maybe.

Nursing Tug of War

Why on earth should there be any form of rivalry between nurses? We are sisters not by blood, but by the very fabric that holds us together. The thread that binds us is our universal code of togetherness woven by our shared experience. Our untold struggles that only we have journeyed should unite us. Our uniqueness from the rest of the world's professions should bring us together. We are a sect unlike any other, preceded by great nurses who paved the way that we may stand as professionals. Together, we uphold and live by the same sacrificial and honorable mantra that most men will not venture into. To each other we owe respect, not petty rivalries.

The irony is that each shift has a preconceived notion of the other. For night nurses it is that they will never be busy and the day shift left their patients so perfect that they will have nothing to do to occupy their time. However, no one is perfect, because moments after shift report is over, untoward events start happening. The night nurse's patients begin to sundown, predicting the path we are about to endure. Next, the night nurse discovers that there is a patient not breathing well on the step down unit who will be making their acquaintance soon. Of course, the respiratory department has now departed. Moments later, the nurse is told she is about to receive a patient who has just been intubated post resuscitation. On arrival they come with feces pasted all over their bottom, vomitus pooled around their endotracheal tube, and a swollen arm from a faulty intravenous line, with no nursing assistant. The only thoughts that continue penetrating her mind are the quotes of the last nurse during report who said "Everything's done for you—you'll have nothing to do." Honestly, how can they say that? This is a field that is highly unpredictable and all those nurses should remember that the unexpected could happen at any time. For the day nurses, the whole world assumes that they have so much extra help, when in actuality there may be lots of extra staff, but they are not always assisting the nurses.

So who really has your back, fellow nurses, when shit hits the fan? We admire your strength when you're bombarded with multiple outpatient/inpatient procedures and you handle it all with such ease. On that note, remember this next time you begin your shift complaining about the previous staff leaving the area untidy. When the incoming shift notices a not-so-perfect counter top or the mile-long telemetry strip that's now resting on the floor, there should be no judgment. Rather, try looking around and notice that the patients are alive and stable. Remember, at the end of the day we are all playing on the same team. United we stand!

Chapter 6

Social Injustice

Success is measured not by what we are able to accomplish but by the many hurdles we overcome on our journey to succeed.

We all have the image of the nurse donned in pure white, with a perfectly proportioned hat atop a perfectly shaped bun, welcomed by patients. Imagine that white, pristine uniform covering awareness of dark stories yet untold. That vision of the perfect and untouchable angel floating into the room of happy and grateful patients no longer exists. Rather, the grateful patient has over the years evolved into an all-knowing authoritarian.

Whoever imagined that a nurse who strives to uphold every life as sacred would encounter prejudice because of the color of her skin? It's unbelievable, but some, whose lives have been spared due not only to divine intervention but by hands a shade darker than theirs, are often the bigots. At times it is subtle, and many times very blatant. It is an insidious plague that is deeply rooted in many and shows its ugly head even at the point when life is at its frailest. Ignorance must be exposed and in the process of that, may it enlighten the minds of many to change. To those nurses who have been the victims of such hatred, know that you are not alone. Stand tall in your mission to save lives and do not be deterred by ignorance, which is as burdensome as any ailment. Eventually, the flower that thrives in a hostile environment will stand, despite what storms may come.

One story that comes to mind is of the patient who called the nurse every few minutes of her shift. The urgent repetitive calls were not for emergencies, mind you. They were in fact deliberate calls to see how far the nurse's limit of patience could be tested. Why? Sadly, it was done as a way to find a reason to raise the claim of insubordination against her. A patient did exactly that. After responding diligently to all his calls, the nurse was caught up in an emergency when another call came through. Without further ado she alerted the patient she would be a few minutes longer.

Soon after, the nurse returned to the patient's room to find a horrific scene before her. Picture this--feces smeared all over the patient's bed, along with every square inch of the floor. A central venous catheter, triple lumen might we add, had been pulled out and flung across the room with droplets of blood everywhere. The response of this very alert and oriented patient may shock you. "You didn't come fast enough!" He said it with an intensity of hatred that gave her chills down her spine. In addition, he mumbled the racial slur "Ni**er!" What would you do? What could you do? That same nurse reported the scenario later to her supervisor, who quickly brushed it off, minimizing an event that has had lasting effect on that nurse to the present day. Why? Fear of losing the patient's money, fear of what managed care would say, fear of challenging the bigot—one or all and more reasons exist, none of them good ones. Instead, that patient was treated like a king after this so-called traumatic experience. It is a shameful and telling aspect of casting a blind eye in hospital management.

Another situation we must describe occurred when a nurse received a report from the outgoing shift who gave rave reviews about the patient she would be receiving. How very polite and quiet the patient was, and more importantly, barely a word was heard from that person for the whole shift. The nurse giving the report continued to compliment this "perfect patient" who is about to be graciously handed over. The outgoing nurse reiterated how sweet this patient was. The only word that this patient uttered was a constant thank you. The outgoing shift staff concluded by saying that the patient rarely rang the call bell and was very knowledgeable about their current plan of care. These beautiful sentiments unfortunately changed when the African American nurse walked into the patient's room to introduce herself. She saw the look of annoyance on the patient's face. At times the patient and their families continued to gaze past that nurse in an exaggerated manner as if they had been ambushed and could not find an escape route. Perhaps they were hoping that it was some dream that they would be awakened from. Or, that there was a mistake somewhere and their "real nurse" will walk in any minute.

At times when the patient has ascertained that they are, for a better word, stuck with that particular nurse, the nurse's life becomes a living hell. That "star patient" now becomes a very demanding, condescending monster who treats her as less than a slave. Suddenly, that nurse becomes the hunted in the pursuit of saving the precious life of someone who has no value for hers. It's not over yet. The nightmare has begun as the nurse graciously answers his frequent bell rings. After patiently responding to all his needs and questions, (which sets her back from her other responsibilities) the nurse dares attempt to exit the room, only for the patient to call her right back.

The allegedly very knowledgeable patient who is cognizant about their plan of care now begins an interrogation about everything, including his test results from long ago, beginning with the mechanism of the action of meds he has taken for a lifetime, with all its side effects and interactions. This is done often enough so that the patient can write a "dissertation" regarding the treatment they received. Every chance they get they accuse that nurse of not knowing what they are doing. Then, after the nurse has patiently explained every question in good faith, he further adds "Did you give me my right meds?" She wants to say, "Yes sir, including the soap suds enema I'm about to instill right up your ass!"

Other patients use a variety of offending words and suddenly nothing makes them happy. Their pain which has been under control for the past few days becomes unbearable when that nurse with the "dark skin" takes them over as a patient, and suddenly their needs aren't being addressed at all. They demand a call be placed to the physician and that they get more pain medicine. Or, their new working IV with no complications suddenly becomes uncomfortable and they want it changed. Why would anyone want pain inflicted on them needlessly? All these and more "orders" are given in a very condescending manner. These patients will refuse to call the nurse by her rightful name. She may not be called nurse, hey or Miss— instead her name will be the look of disappointment on the patient's face. The patient may throw out a name that is totally opposite and which simply has no resemblance to the nurse's actual name. Ironically, a nurse a few shades lighter walks in and suddenly she is magically greeted with a smile and addressed by her proper name for the entirety of her shift.

In a very patronizing manner, the nurse can be asked at the end of her very painful shift to come hold the urinal one last time while flatulence is released in her face as a parting gift. She yet again holds her head high against the wrongful acts of discrimination.

There is also the patient who, after the nurse has spent weeks battling to save his life, recovers due to her diligent expertise and care. The magical words that they utter are not where are they or how long have they been in the hospital but, "Are you from around here?" Each and every nurse wishes at one point in her career they can actually say what they are really thinking:

-No, I'm from Mars.

-How long have you been a nurse?

-Long enough to know better.

-You have an accent?

-No shit, Sherlock, so do you.

-Is that your real hair?

-It is now, paid in full.

It is rude to ask if someone's hair is real or not, or any other part of them. A simple compliment would suffice. Nurses don't ask if a patient has had her breasts augmented when it is blatantly obvious.

Bigotry still exists today, my friends, even when life lies in the balance. When darkness falls there is no distinction in creed or color. The very blood that runs through our veins has the same hue and consistency. We all journey but for a brief period and death knows no race. Neither does the threat of disease favor a few because of their complexion. When a lifesaving transfusion brings back a patient from death's door they have no idea from whence their saving grace cometh.

Chapter 7

Healing Hands

To be in the service of humanity, no matter how you see it, is a spiritual matter whether it is acknowledged or not. Nursing has many rewards. It is these rewards that maintain our equilibrium and bring a sense of peace to our vocation. To serve those who are helpless, to give comfort to the suffering, to heal with our hands— the list goes on and on. These are the values that every nurse holds. A nurse takes charge of the patient's entire being, both physical, mental, and emotional.

Some nurses begin their day visiting a house of worship, sitting at times in silence before a higher power, placing every patient that they will encounter in his or her hands. In the silence of their hearts, they pray for the health and recovery of their patients, placing their shift under divine guidance. Still, many pray specific chaplets or novenas for their patients. One such is the Divine Mercy prayer that is prayed over the sick in a variety of ways, for the vented patient on the brink of terminal extubation, behind closed curtains away from the eyes of colleagues or families alike, or for the patient who after a successful surgery is now well and is close to being discharged. Projecting a spirit of wellness in our thoughts, surrounding our hospitals with the fire of divine love, performing CPR on a patient who is deceased, fighting the hands of death, all of this is in itself is a spiritual act of mercy. *Whatsoever you do to the least of my brothers that you do unto me*.... Nurses live this song, well known by many, in all kinds of ways.

When one is faced with the fragility of life there is a feeling of fear that the presence of a nurse can soothe away. Many sick people struggle at the end of their lives with emotional conflicts that nurses always have an ear for, whether it is the need to forgive or to be forgiven. When all hope seems to be lost, it is the nurse who helps the patient find meaning in his or her life.

We have been known to pray with the patients as their souls ascend from their bodies. Nurses remain with their patients long before families arrive holding their hands. We say go well, rest in peace. May this medicine give you comfort in your last moments. You are not alone, we are here with you. Many times nurses do this after waiting for family members who cannot be present when the patient's journey is at its end.

During post mortem care (yes, nurses are also the morticians), we prepare their bodies for the morgue with dignity. Cleansing the body that once stood amidst the living, seeing them not merely as a patient, but who they really were, a mother or father to someone, grandparents, teachers, sons and daughters. Words of peace are spoken to the spirit of the deceased in thought and deed. Finally, we are at times the last to gently close their eyes for their journey's end where there will be no pain or disease. To be a part of the sacredness of life in all its stages, even death, is an experience that is very humbling and life-changing.

At such times there is nothing medical science can provide. On other occasions it is the futility and hopelessness of a case that propels us to seek a higher power. One such experience a nurse had was that of a young man whose liver failed as a result of Hepatitis. This man had a long course of pain and agony due to his condition. He had been in and out of the hospital with complications, and finally after many years on a waiting list for a transplant, he received one, only to face rejection. Sadly, he received a second transplant, which also was on the verge of failing. His case was rendered futile until his primary nurse went on a mission of prayer and supplication on his behalf. When all else seemed lost he came through. Shortly after receiving his new liver, he returned home happy, not knowing that his nurse had prayed for him every waking hour.

There are those patients, on the other hand, who remain in our psyche many years after caring for them. Some stories are so tragic that they leave a mark on our own lives and practice. There once was an elderly couple that had been married sixty years. They were the light of life to each other. Blissfully happy after all those years, they remained inseparable. This couple still had a spark in their eyes for each other. They did not behave like the typical seventy-eight and seventy nine-year-olds. In fact, they had planned on taking a winter sabbatical. She laughed animatedly as she shared their plans. This break would give them a warm tropical winter, rather than the usual chilly ones they had been accustomed to. Prior to their planning, the Mrs. began having issues with her Diverticulitis. Unfortunately, many people suffer with this condition and can describe the long-term effects it can cause. Rather than take the chance having any issues while being two thousand miles away from her surgeon, she decided to electively have her surgery sooner rather than later. That following week, she was prepped and ready to go. The surgery seemed uneventful despite the low blood pressure in recovery and the time it took to wake up. Everything appeared to go as planned. Her darling devoted husband stayed with her the entire day and soon as she was stable he went home to get some rest.

Later that evening, she seemed slightly off. She couldn't put her finger on it and neither could her doctor. The odd thing was that around nine-thirty at night, her worried husband could not sleep due to her absence. He explained he felt unsettled and needed to kiss her goodnight as he had done for the past sixty years of their marriage. After escorting him out, the nurse returned to give his wife her evening meds. Less than five minutes of chatting transpired regarding her concerns about her husband driving home with his poor night vision. Then it happened. Within seconds, she grabbed her chest while a light hue of blue overtook her complexion. Her heart rhythm went into a lethal arrhythmia. All efforts to save her proved ineffective and she eventually lost her battle. It was absolutely heartbreaking. It was almost as if the husband knew and he had to see her one last time.

You see, nurses are there when no one else is. Their hearts break right along with their patients and their families. They carry those stories in their hearts and try to find some form of solace. They also relive every step over and over again holding the memory of that patient. In the business of saving lives, nurses wonder whether the patient's death had to do with something they missed. In some cases, no matter what our efforts may be, no amount of intervention will bring the patient back.

Chapter 8

TRIBUTES TO NURSES

Emergency room nurses, we thank you for tolerating those who decide to sample or simply indulge in Ecstasy for enhanced aphrodisiac effect that leads them to your Emergency room at four a.m. with self-induced seizures. Or the college student who goes overboard drinking at their first fraternity party and shows up unconscious for you to consistently prevent them from aspirating their vomit. What about the patient with tooth pain that presents asking for Dilaudid, because it worked so great the last time their tooth pain flared up? Let's not forget that drunk guy the police brought in for blood sampling who won't stop slurring and drooling in your face. More often the elderly patients from the nursing homes who just didn't seem right would have a core temperature of one hundred four! Don't forget to initiate that sepsis protocol. Or, what about the gentleman who decided to place a dumbbell weight around the base of his penis after doing cocaine and masturbating, which led him to pass out with that same weight now needing to be surgically removed.

We thank you!

Medical surgical nurses, we thank you for tolerating having to push your life-sized computer to the rooms of your seven patients at a steady pace. We appreciate your craftiness in gathering all of your confused patients in front of the nursing station to prevent falls, delivering prune juice to all your bowel-fixated patients, making endless trips to your pixis machines for your patients who know the exact time they are due for more narcotics, for putting up with the certified nursing assistant who tells you how to fix the patients draw sheet, for getting so many admissions you forget their names and view them as diseases, and worse; discover four out of five of your patients are in isolation. Your charge nurse talks the entire shift while critiquing your every move. Even when you get floated to the ICU or ER you still maintain your professionalism.

We thank you!

Rehab nurses, we thank you for tolerating the patient who insists on a shower at the end of your shift, although when you had free time, your offer was repeatedly rejected. For dealing with the hordes of documentation required of you. For attempting to instill rehabilitation in a confused patient. And mostly for not flipping out when they float you to the medical surgical floor!

We thank you!

Intensive care nurses, thank you for being the rock stars that you are. We appreciate your assessment skills first and foremost. We appreciate your tolerating those annoying stat transfers from every unit known to man that have left out most of the pertinent information in the report. For dealing with your morning doctors rounds and your outpatient procedures. For getting partners that sit and text while you're assisting with intubation. For not punching someone in the face when they float you to the emergency room or the medical surgical floors. For drawing the morning labs while the lab tech stares you down. For being everyone's backup, but when you need it, no one comes. For being forced to become the Ebola specialist when management decides the ICU team will accept and care for any Ebola patient that will be admitted.

We thank you!

Obstetric nurses, we thank you for your tolerance of the patient in labor for ten hours. For dealing with the variety of mothers, some too young, some neglectful, addicts, pristine moms that need their beauty sleep after only bonding with their baby for an hour. For teaching the mothers nipple care so they don't feel like their nipples are about to fall off. For your readiness to adapt to all birth wishes and to stand strong when the worst outcome presents itself.

We thank you!

Recovery room nurses, we thank you for your perseverance in accommodating the patient who after having a serious bowel surgery opens their eyes and insists on having their partial dentures cleaned and put back in their mouths. For recovering a teenager who insists on requesting all the don'ts in post-operative care like food, water—the list goes on and on. For assisting the patient who takes a turn for the worse and requires quick intervention.

We thank you!

School nurses, we thank you. Whether it's primary, middle, or high school, you take on a tough bunch on a daily basis. It's a unique world with which we are unfamiliar. From the little scrapes on the knees, stomach aches, fevers, or simply to escape an unwanted subject, the school nurse is where the students go. Sometimes just your presence can be a nurturing substitute to comfort a kindergartener who misses his or her parent. In any case, we thank you not only for your patience but your devotion to the children. Mostly, we envy your summers off!

We thank you!

To all nursing home staff, we thank you. We appreciate all your hard work and care provided on an individual basis, considering the daily routines of your residents. It's a job that doesn't pay as well as it should, either. The amount of work done by the certified nursing assistant is not only commendable but should be recognized more. The workload of the morning "get ups" to the meals--the tasks are endless. These residents are living their final chapter out in their new all-too-temporary "home" and the importance of maintaining the resident's dignity is of the utmost importance.

We thank you!

Praise to the correctional nurses for showing compassion to a murderer, child molester, and rapist, among many. We value your courage and fortitude as you begin your day, entering a dungeon filled with society's most hardened criminals. Yet you return each and every day to serve humanity at its worst, including those who offer a myriad of imaginary symptoms to gain a temporary fix. You go above and beyond to obtain contraband from the vilest of forms.

We thank you!

Bravo to the transplant nurses. You are the glue that holds the patient together when their bodily organs can no longer sustain them, specifically, the liver transplant patients who present with liver failure. Good old liver, garbage disposal of all things unwanted, goes awry and all hell breaks loose. We appreciate your stamina as you respond appropriately to the failing organ and all that it implies. The marred coagulation factors sends patients vomiting blood even when the nurse isn't prepared for it—yet you are there to "catch it." You are special indeed. In the end, not all transplants are successful, and you are the patient's emotional support, giving hope to the hopeless.

We thank you!

Praise for the Neonatal Intensive Care Nurses. Your healing touch is the foundation of their recovery, the fragile little angels, whose every milestone to survival can become a struggle that only the NICU nurse can relate to. They are too weak to fight for their new life, so the NICU nurse stands vigilant, giving them much needed affection, leading the fight to keep little babies alive, and they never underestimate the power these precious ones hold, treating each child with open arms, regardless of their underlining social or medical attributes.

We thank you!

Oncology nurses, we thank you for the selfless acts you provide that go above and beyond your job description. No job can prepare your emotions for the unpredictable outcomes. Your role in guiding your patients through the emotional challenges and stages is praiseworthy. Not all of us could withstand the emotional load of your job on a daily basis. Each and every case comes with increased grief, requiring strong interpersonal skills and compassion from you. You continue to provide support throughout that patient's journey. Unfortunately, not all have positive outcomes.

We thank you!

The specialties of nursing are endless and we salute you all, for your dedication and professionalism at all times, no matter the circumstances. You truly are a remarkable bunch of men and women. It takes a special kind of person to do what we do. Mightier than any emergent disease is the hand that can repair what is broken. It is the neutralizing remedy for many ailments, the counteragent to many poisons. Without the nurse, life when it is at its most trying moment, can be hoisted, but not uplifted. We stand at the helm of life's beginning and at its end rowing precious lives to the shore of wellness. **The world, with all its wounds may be mended, but the ability to heal and repair what is seen and unseen is in the power of a good nurse.**

At the end of the day, it's all about our patients and the care they receive. This is why we all became nurses—to uphold the standard we have today. In the words of Florence Nightingale;

"I solemnly pledge myself before God and in the presence of this assembly, to pass my life in purity and to practice my profession faithfully. I will abstain from whatever is deleterious and

mischievous, and will not take or knowingly administer any harmful drug. I will do all in my power to maintain and elevate the standard of my profession, and will hold in all confidence all personal matters committed to my keeping and all family affairs coming to my knowledge in the practice of my calling. With loyalty will I endeavor to aid the physician in his work, and devote myself to the welfare of those committed to my care".

This beautiful and heartfelt rendition by our predecessor applies not only to those mentioned but to our young and to each other.

You were the warm hands that welcomed me into this world.
There you stood by my side when my journey was at its final
end
With your beautiful spirit you encouraged my first breath.
Bringing forth my first cry that became my voice.
When I couldn't find words you spoke for me.
My tears, you wiped away with your kindness
You saw the real me underneath the diagnosis,
Beneath the emaciated person that I had become.
You found me and beckoned the very life within me to
flourish.
You are earthly angels that walk this earth giving healing
with your powerful touch.

Written by Stella Joseph and Helen

About the Authors

We are registered nurses who have been in this profession for over fifteen years. We honestly have seen it all and at times wish we hadn't. The vast majority of our lives is spent multitasking our careers and raising our children while bringing to light our passion for writing. Through our combined experience, we have worked in the emergency room, intensive care unit, medical surgical floor, transplant unit, home care, corrections, psychiatric, nursing home, and have cared for pediatric patients as well. Our varied clinical experiences give us the impetus to shed a little light on what we do as nurses. The ability to participate in healing and to witness the difference we make in many lives is what drives us. Our shared passion for nursing deepens each day as we join forces with our fellow nurses in combatting emerging diseases with sacrifice and grace.

www.ingramcontent.com/pod-product-compliance
Lightning Source LLC
Chambersburg PA
CBHW051816170526
45167CB00005B/2044

9781505659153